GLUTEN FREE GUT HEALTH COOKBOOK

Healthy Gluten-Free Recipes for Gut Vitality

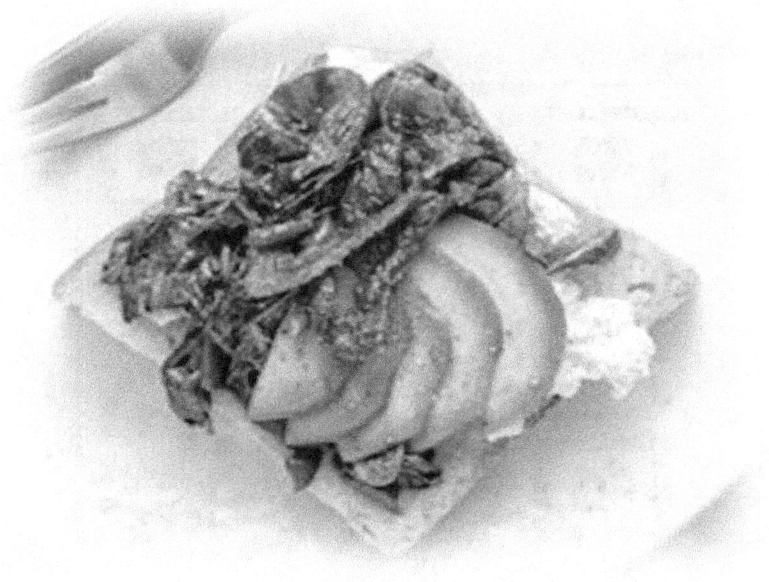

CHRISTIANA WHITE

GAIN ACCESS TO MORE BOOKS

TABLE OF CONTENTS.

INTRODUCTION

Every kitchen contains the power to transform lives, one meal at a time. "The Gluten Free Gut Health Cookbook" is more than simply a compilation of recipes; it's a fresh start for individuals dealing with gut health difficulties. This book is a witness to the healing journeys of numerous people who have found consolation inside its pages.

Imagine Anna's relief, who was once doubled over in anguish from bloating but now begins her days with a smile owing to the calming quinoa porridge and vivid salads.

Consider John, who said goodbye to the cloudy head and joint pain that hampered his steps, and is now experiencing clarity and ease with each spoonful of bone broth and bite of almond flour muffins. Their stories are just a few examples of how the promise of a gluten-free route to wellbeing has improved many people's lives.

This cookbook is more than just a guide; it's a companion for individuals looking for relief from the symptoms of gluten intolerance. It's a beacon of hope for anyone looking to restore their health and energy. Each recipe is a celebration of flavor, precisely prepared to nourish the body and thrill the senses while adhering to the strictest gluten-free guidelines.

As you turn each page, you'll learn not only how to make delicious, gut-friendly meals, but also how to enjoy and appreciate nature's simple, healthful ingredients. This book invites you to go on a journey of healing, to discover the limitless possibilities of a gluten-free diet, and to join the ranks of others who have already changed their lives.

"The Gluten Free Gut Health Cookbook" is more than simply a purchase; it's an investment in health, a commitment to well-being, and a step toward a happier, more vibrant existence. Welcome to a world where every meal presents an opportunity to heal, thrive, and enjoy the richness of a gluten-free diet that actually nourishes from within.

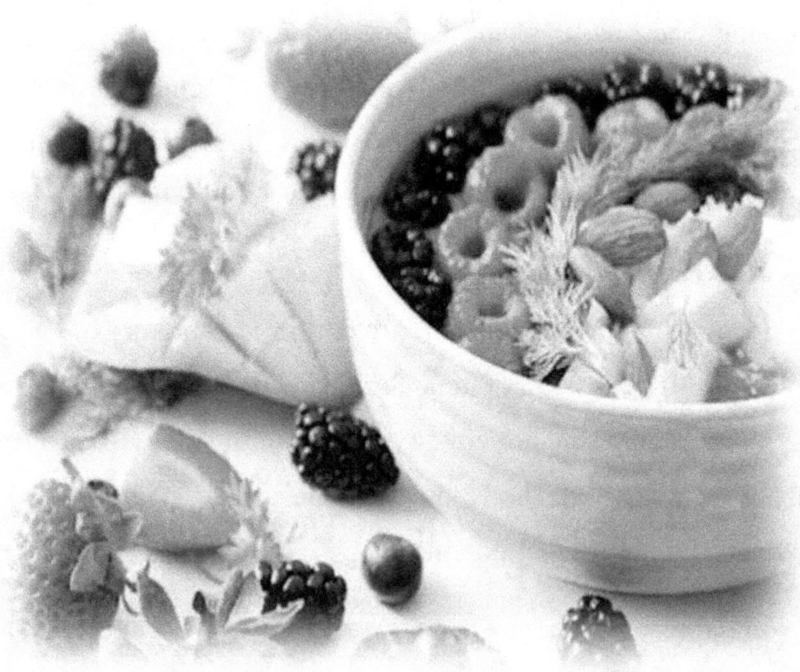

CHAPTER 1

Understanding the Gluten-free Gut Health Diet

The gluten-free gut health diet aims to promote a healthy digestive system by removing gluten, a protein present in wheat, barley and rye.

This diet is especially good for people who have gluten-related conditions such as celiac disease or non-celiac gluten sensitivity. Even people who have not been diagnosed with a disease may benefit from a gluten-free diet.

Importance of Gut Health

The gut, commonly known as the gastrointestinal tract, is a complex and intriguing ecosystem teeming with billions of creatures like bacteria, fungi, and viruses. The gut microbiome is a varied community that plays an important role in general health.

- Digestion and nutrient absorption: The gut microbiota degrades food, allowing humans to acquire vital nutrients.
- Immune function: A healthy gut microbiota trains the immune system to distinguish between safe chemicals and hazardous infections.

- Mood and mental health: There is mounting research relating gut health to psychological well-being.
- Overall health: Gut health has been related to a variety of health issues, including obesity, diabetes, heart disease, and skin health.

When the gut microbiota is balanced, it performs optimally. However, variables such as nutrition, stress, and drugs can disrupt the delicate balance, resulting in gut dysbiosis, a condition in which harmful bacteria outnumber helpful bacteria. This imbalance can cause digestive troubles, inflammation, and other health problems.

How Gluten Affects the Gut

Gluten causes an autoimmune response in patients with celiac disease. When they consume gluten, their immune system wrongly assaults the lining of the small intestine, causing inflammation and injury. This damage reduces nutrient absorption and causes a variety of digestive and health difficulties.

Non-celiac gluten sensitivity does not include an immunological response, although some people still report gastrointestinal pain after eating gluten. Symptoms may include bloating, gas, diarrhea, and abdominal pain. These symptoms are most likely caused by gluten's influence on the gut lining and the alteration of the gut microbiota.

Gluten can cause stomach problems even in those who have not been diagnosed with gluten sensitivity. Gluten has been linked in studies to increased intestinal permeability, often known as leaky gut. This can cause inflammation and the introduction of undesirable substances into the bloodstream.

People with celiac disease see dramatic improvements in gut health after eliminating gluten from their diet. The inflammation subsides, allowing the small intestine to repair and absorb nutrients more efficiently. Similarly, persons with non-celiac gluten sensitivity may notice that their stomach symptoms improve or go entirely after following a gluten-free diet.

While research is ongoing, there is growing evidence that a gluten-free diet can help some people have a better gut microbiota. Even those who have not been diagnosed with gluten-related diseases may benefit from improved gut health.

CHAPTER 2

Identifying Gluten-Containing Foods

Knowing where gluten hides is essential for a healthy gluten-free gut health diet. Here's a list of typical gluten-containing foods and hidden sources to look out for.

Obvious Gluten Sources:

- Grains: wheat (all types), barley, rye, spelt, triticale (a wheat-rye hybrid).

- Baked goods include bread, spaghetti, crackers, cookies, cakes, pastries, muffins, and cereals (unless clearly labelled gluten-free).

- Processed foods include fried or battered meats, processed snacks (chips, pretzels, etc.), condiments (soy sauce, teriyaki sauce, salad dressings), soups, sauces, and beer.

Hidden Gluten Sources:

- Modified Food Starches: These are sourced from wheat and may show on ingredient lists as wheat starch, modified wheat starch, or hydrolysed wheat protein.

- Malt is commonly found in malted milk products, malt vinegar, and several breakfast cereals.

- Barley: Found in malt used to make beer and several processed foods.

- Oats: Although oats are inherently gluten-free, they can quickly get contaminated with wheat during processing. To ensure safety, choose certified gluten-free oats.
- Cross-Contamination: Avoid using utensils, cookware, or surfaces that have been in touch with gluten-containing meals.

Tips to Identify Gluten:

- Always read labels carefully: Look for any of the gluten-containing cereals or derivatives specified on the ingredient list. Look for labels that clearly say "gluten-free."
- "May Contain" Disclaimer: There is a potential of gluten contamination during processing. If you are severely sensitive, exercise cautious or avoid using these products.
- Download Gluten-Free Apps: There are several apps that can help you scan barcodes and identify gluten-containing substances.

Essential Gluten-Free Ingredients

The good news is that there are many naturally gluten-free ingredients available to make delicious and healthful meals. Here are some gluten-free pantry staples:

- Gluten-free grains: quinoa, brown rice, white rice, black rice, wild rice, millet, sorghum, amaranth, and buckwheat (not technically wheat).

- Starchy vegetables include potatoes, sweet potatoes, butternut squash, and corn (depending on sensitivity).

- Gluten-free flours include almond flour, coconut flour, chickpea flour (gram flour), oat flour (certified gluten-free), tapioca flour, and brown rice flour.

- Protein sources: lean meats, poultry, fish, seafood, legumes (beans, lentils, chickpeas), tofu, tempeh.

- Oils and fats: olive, avocado, coconut, almonds (if tolerated), seeds.

- Fruits and veggies: Fill your kitchen with a variety of fruits and veggies for vitamins, minerals, and fiber.

Tips for Gluten-Free Culinary Success

Going gluten-free should not imply compromising flavor or diversity! Here are some practical strategies to improve your gluten-free cooking:

- Master Gluten-Free Flours: Experiment with various gluten-free flours to determine which mixes work best for specific recipes. Because each flour has distinct properties, a one-to-one substitution with wheat flour may not always be effective.

- Use Natural Binders: Use flaxseed meal, chia seeds, or eggs as binders to keep your gluten-free baked goods together.

- Xanthan Gum is Your Friend: This popular gluten-free baking ingredient mimics the elasticity that gluten provides in dough.

- Be Creative with Thickening Agents: Arrowroot powder, cornstarch, and tapioca flour are excellent substitutes for wheat flour as a thickener in soups and sauces.

- Investigate Alternative Grains: Enjoy the distinct Flavors and textures of gluten-free grains such as quinoa, brown rice, and sorghum.

- Don't Forget Flavor Boosters: Use herbs, spices, citrus zest, and extracts to add depth and complexity to your gluten-free recipes.

- Invest in a Good Blender: A high-powered blender can be extremely useful for making smooth batters, dips, sauces, and even nut butters.
- Become Certified: When buying pre-made mixes or baked goods, look for the certified gluten-free label to ensure safety.

With a little planning and these helpful hints, you can confidently navigate the world of gluten-free cooking and prepare delicious meals that support your gut health.

CHAPTER 3

Breakfasts to Begin Your Day Right

Quinoa Porridge and Mixed Berries

- ***Servings: Two.***
- ***Prep time: 5 minutes.***
- ***Cook time: 15 minutes.***

Ingredients:

- 1 cup washed quinoa.
- Two glasses of almond milk.
- One cup mixed berry.
- 2 tablespoons honey or maple syrup.
- 1 teaspoon of vanilla extract.
- A pinch of salt.

Instructions:

- In a saucepan, combine quinoa, almond milk, and a teaspoon of salt. Bring to a boil.
- Reduce the heat to low, cover, and simmer for 15 minutes.
- Remove from heat and cover for 5 minutes.
- Mix in the vanilla extract and honey or maple syrup.
- Serve hot, topped with mixed berries.

<u>*Buckwheat Pancakes with Maple Syrup*</u>

- *Serves: 4*
- *Prep time: 10 minutes.*
- *Cook time: 20 minutes.*

Ingredients:

- One cup buckwheat flour.
- One tablespoon of baking powder.
- 1/4 teaspoon salt.
- One cup of almond milk.
- 1 egg (or flax egg for the vegan version).
- 2 tablespoons melted coconut oil.
- Maple syrup to serve.

Instructions:

- In a bowl, combine the buckwheat flour, baking powder, and salt.
- In a separate bowl, whisk together the almond milk, egg, and coconut oil.
- Mix the wet and dry ingredients until smooth.
- Heat a nonstick pan over medium heat, then pour 1/4 cup batter for each pancake.
- Cook until bubbles appear on the surface, then turn and finish until golden brown.
- Serve with maple syrup.

Chia Seed Pudding with Almond Milk

- *Servings: Two.*
- *Prep time: 5 minutes.*
- *Rest time: four hours or overnight.*

Ingredients:

- 1/4 cup of chia seeds.
- One cup of almond milk.
- One tablespoon maple syrup.
- 1/2 teaspoon vanilla extract.

Instructions:

- In a bowl, combine the almond milk, maple syrup, and vanilla essence.
- Add the chia seeds and stir thoroughly.
- Let the mixture sit for 5 minutes before stirring again.
- Cover and chill for at least 4 hours, preferably overnight.
- Stir before serving, and add more almond milk as needed for the appropriate consistency.

Smoothie Bowl: Spinach, Avocado, and Banana

- *Serves: 1*
- *Prep time: 5 minutes.*

Ingredients:

- One ripe banana.
- One-half avocado
- One cup of fresh spinach.
- One-half cup almond milk
- Toppings: sliced fruits, nuts and seeds.

Instructions:

- Blend the banana, avocado, spinach, and almond milk until smooth.
- Pour into a bowl and top with your preferred toppings.

Amaranth and Almond Milk Breakfast Bake.

- *Serves: 4*
- *Prep time: 10 minutes.*
- *Cook time: 30 minutes.*

Ingredients:

- One cup amaranth.
- Two glasses of almond milk.
- 1/4 cup maple syrup.
- 1/2 teaspoon cinnamon.
- 1/4 cup chopped almonds.

Instructions:

- Preheat the oven to 350°F (175° C).
- In a baking dish, mix together amaranth, almond milk, maple syrup, and cinnamon.
- Bake for 30 minutes, until the liquid has been absorbed.
- Finish with chopped almonds and serve warm.

Gluten-Free Oats with Cinnamon and Apples.

- *Servings: Two.*
- *Prep time: 5 minutes.*
- *Cooking Time: 10 minutes.*

Ingredients:

- One cup gluten-free rolled oats.
- 2 cups water or almond milk.
- One apple, diced
- One teaspoon of cinnamon.
- Add honey or maple syrup to taste.

Instructions:

- In a saucepan, heat water or almond milk until it boils.
- Add oats and decrease heat to a simmer.
- Cook 10 minutes, stirring occasionally.
- Stir in the diced apples and cinnamon.
- Finish with a drizzle of honey or maple syrup.

Baked Sweet Potatoes with Yogurt and Nuts.

- *Servings: Two.*
- *Prep time: 5 minutes.*
- *Cook time: 45 minutes.*

Ingredients:

• Two medium sweet potatoes.

• 1/2 cup Greek yogurt (or coconut yogurt if dairy-free).

• 1/4 cup mixed nuts, chopped

• Add honey or maple syrup to taste.

Instructions:

- Preheat the oven to 400°F (200° C).
- Pierce the sweet potatoes with a fork and bake for 45 minutes, or until soft.
- Cut the sweet potatoes open and top with yogurt and almonds.
- Drizzle with honey or maple syrup before serving.

Savory Vegetable Muffins

- *Servings: 12 muffins.*
- *Prep time: 15 minutes.*
- *Cook time: 25 minutes.*

Ingredients:

- 2 cups gluten-free flour mixture.
- One tablespoon of baking powder.
- 1/2 teaspoon salt.
- One cup of almond milk.
- One-quarter cup olive oil
- Two eggs (or flax eggs for the vegan option).
- 1 cup finely chopped mixed vegetables.

Instructions:

- Preheat the oven to 350°F/175°C and butter a muffin tray.
- In a bowl, combine the flour, baking powder, and salt.
- In another bowl, combine almond milk, oil, and eggs.
- Mix the wet and dry ingredients, then fold in the vegetables.
- Scoop the batter into muffin cups and bake for 25 minutes, or until a toothpick comes out clean.

Coconut Yogurt with Gluten-Free Granola

- *Servings: Two*
- *Prep time: 5 minutes.*

Ingredients:

- One cup of coconut yogurt.
- 1/2 cup of gluten-free granola
- Fresh fruits as topping

Instructions:

- Spoon coconut yogurt into bowls.
- Sprinkle with gluten-free granola and fresh fruit.

Egg White Omelette with Spinach and Mushroom

- *Serves: 1*
- *Prep time: 5 minutes.*
- *Cooking Time: 10 minutes.*

Ingredients:

- Three egg whites.
- 1/2 cup chopped spinach.
- 1/4 cup sliced mushrooms.
- Add salt and pepper to taste.

- One tablespoon olive oil.

Instructions:

- Heat olive oil in a nonstick skillet over medium heat.
- Sauté the mushrooms until browned, then add the spinach and simmer until wilted.
- Whisk egg whites with salt and pepper before pouring over the vegetables.
- Cook the omelette until the eggs are set, then fold in half and serve.

CHAPTER 4

Nutritious And Delicious Lunches

Quinoa Salad with Roasted Vegetables.

- *Serves: 4*
- *Prep time: 15 minutes.*
- *Cook time: 30 minutes.*

Ingredients:

- One cup quinoa.
- Two glasses of water.
- 1 bell pepper, diced
- 1 zucchini, diced
- One carrot, chopped
- One tablespoon of olive oil.
- Add salt and pepper to taste.
- Two teaspoons of balsamic vinegar.

Instructions:

- Preheat your oven to 400°F (200°C).
- Rinse the quinoa in cool water and drain.

- In a saucepan, heat 2 cups of water till boiling. Add the quinoa, reduce the heat to low, cover, and cook for 15 minutes.
- While the quinoa cooks, combine the diced vegetables with olive oil, salt, and pepper.
- Place the vegetables on a baking sheet and roast for 20 minutes until soft.
- Fluff the cooked quinoa with a fork and mix in the roasted vegetables.
- Toss with balsamic vinegar and serve.

Buckwheat Soba Noodle Salad.

- *Serves: 4*
- *Prep time: 10 minutes.*
- *Cook time: 5 minutes.*

Ingredients:

- 8 ounces buckwheat soba noodles.
- 1 cucumber julienned
- 1 red bell pepper, thinly sliced
- One-quarter cup rice vinegar
- Two tablespoons of tamari (gluten-free soy sauce).
- One tablespoon of sesame oil.

- One teaspoon of honey.
- Sesame seeds as garnish

Instructions:

- Cook the soba noodles according to the package directions, then rinse with cold water and drain.
- In a large bowl, combine the noodles, cucumber, and bell pepper.
- In a small bowl, combine the rice vinegar, tamari, sesame oil, and honey.
- Pour the dressing over the noodles and toss to coat.
- Sprinkle with sesame seeds and serve chilled.

Grilled Chicken Breast with Avocado and Mango Salsa.

- *Serves: 4*
- *Prep time: 15 minutes.*
- *Cooking Time: 10 minutes.*

Ingredients:

- 4 boneless and skinless chicken breasts.
- Add salt and pepper to taste.
- One ripe mango, diced

- One ripe avocado, chopped

- 1/2 red onion, coarsely chopped

- Juice from 1 lime

- 1 tablespoon of chopped cilantro.

Instructions:

- Preheat the grill to medium-high heat.

- Season the chicken breasts with salt and pepper.

- Grill the chicken for 5 minutes on each side, or until well done.

- In a mixing bowl, combine mango, avocado, red onion, lime juice, and cilantro to make the salsa.

- Serve the grilled chicken topped with fresh salsa.

Lentil Soup with Carrots and Celery

- ***Servings: Six.***
- ***Prep time: 10 minutes.***
- ***Cook time: 40 minutes.***

Ingredients:

- 1 cup of dried lentils, washed

- One tablespoon of olive oil.

- 1 onion, diced

- Two carrots, chopped

- 2 celery stalks, chopped
- Four cups of veggie broth.
- Add salt and pepper to taste.
- One teaspoon thyme.

Instructions:

- Heat the olive oil in a big pot over medium heat.
- Cook the onion, carrots, and celery until softened.
- Combine the lentils, vegetable broth, salt, pepper, and thyme.
- Bring to a boil, then reduce the heat and simmer for 30 minutes, or until the lentils are cooked.
- Serve hot and garnish with fresh herbs if preferred.

Baked Falafel with Tahini Sauce

- *Serves: 4*
- *Prep time: 20 minutes.*
- *Cook time: 30 minutes.*

Ingredients:

- 2 cups canned chickpeas (drained and rinsed)
- 1 onion, chopped
- 2 garlic cloves, minced
- 1/4 cup fresh parsley, chopped

- One teaspoon of ground cumin
- Add salt and pepper to taste.
- Two tablespoons of gluten-free flour.
- 1/4 cup tahini.
- Juice from 1 lemon

Instructions:

- Preheat the oven to 375°F (190°C), then line a baking sheet with parchment paper.
- In a food processor, mix together chickpeas, onion, garlic, parsley, cumin, salt, pepper, and gluten-free flour. Pulse until thoroughly blended but still somewhat lumpy.
- Shape the mixture into tiny patties and set them on the prepared baking sheet.
- Bake for 25–30 minutes, flipping halfway through, until golden and crispy.
- To make the tahini sauce, whisk together tahini and lemon juice, adding water as needed to achieve the appropriate consistency.
- Serve falafel with tahini sauce on top.

<u>Stuffed Bell Peppers with Ground Turkey and Herbs.</u>

- *Serves: 4*
- *Prep time: 15 minutes.*
- *Cook time: 35 minutes.*

Ingredients:

- 4 bell peppers with tops removed and seeded
- One pound of ground turkey
- 1 onion, diced
- 2 garlic cloves, minced
- One cup cooked quinoa.
- One teaspoon of dried oregano.
- One teaspoon of dried basil
- Add salt and pepper to taste.
- 1/2 cup of tomato sauce.

Instructions:

- Preheat the oven to 350°F/175°C.
- Cook ground turkey, onion, and garlic in a pan over medium heat until browned.
- Mix in the cooked quinoa, oregano, basil, salt, pepper, and tomato sauce.

- Stuff the bell peppers with the mixture and place in a baking dish.
- Bake for 30 minutes, or until the peppers are soft and the filling is thoroughly cooked.

Cauliflower Rice Stir-Fry with Mixed Vegetables.

- *Serves: 4*
- *Prep time: 10 minutes.*
- *Cooking Time: 10 minutes.*

Ingredients:

- One head of cauliflower, shredded into rice-sized pieces
- One tablespoon of sesame oil.
- 1 cup mixed veggies (broccoli, carrots, and peas).
- Two tablespoons of tamari (gluten-free soy sauce).
- 1 clove garlic, minced
- One teaspoon of grated ginger.

Instructions:

- Heat the sesame oil in a large skillet over medium heat.
- Cook garlic and ginger until fragrant.
- Stir-fry the cauliflower rice and mixed vegetables for around 5-7 minutes.

- Add tamari and stir-fry until the vegetables are soft and the cauliflower rice is cooked.
- Serve hot.

Spinach And Goat Cheese Frittata

- ***Servings: Six.***
- ***Prep time: 10 minutes.***
- ***Cook time: 20 minutes.***

Ingredients:

- 8 eggs
- Add salt and pepper to taste.
- Two cups of fresh spinach
- 1/2 cup crumbled goat cheese.
- One tablespoon of olive oil.

Instructions:

- Preheat your oven to 375°F (190°C).
- In a bowl, combine the eggs, salt, and pepper.
- Heat the olive oil in an oven-safe skillet over medium heat.
- Add the spinach and simmer until wilted.
- Pour the eggs over the spinach, then sprinkle with goat cheese.

- Place the skillet in the oven and bake for 18-20 minutes, or until the eggs set.

Zucchini Noodles with Pesto and Cherry Tomatoes.

- *Serves: 4*
- *Prep time: 10 minutes.*
- *Cook time: 5 minutes.*

Ingredients:

- 4 medium zucchinis spiralized
- One-half cup pesto
- One cup cherry tomato, halved
- Add salt and pepper to taste.
- Grated Parmesan cheese (for garnish)

Instructions:

- In a large mixing bowl, combine the zucchini noodles and pesto until completely coated.
- Add the cherry tomatoes, salt, and pepper and toss again.
- Serve immediately, topped with Parmesan cheese.

Gluten-Free Tortilla Wraps with Turkey and Spinach.

- _Serves: 4_
- _Prep time: 10 minutes._
- _Cook Time: 0 minutes._

Ingredients:

- Four gluten-free tortillas.
- Eight slices of turkey breast
- Two cups of fresh spinach
- Half-cup chopped carrots
- 1/4 cup hummus.

Instructions:

- Arrange the tortillas on a level surface.
- Spread hummus over each tortilla.
- Place the turkey, spinach, and shredded carrots on top of the hummus.
- Roll the tortillas tightly, then cut in half and serve.

CHAPTER 5

Satisfying Dinners

Grilled Salmon with Lemon and Dill.

- *Serves: 4*
- *Prep time: 10 minutes.*

Ingredients:

- Four salmon fillets.
- 2 tablespoons fresh dill, chopped
- 1 lemon (juice and zest)
- Two teaspoons of olive oil.
- Salt and pepper to taste.

Instructions:

- Preheat the grill to medium-high heat.
- In a small bowl, combine the olive oil, lemon juice, zest, dill, salt, and pepper.
- Brush the mixture onto the salmon fillets.
- Grill the salmon for 3-5 minutes per side, or until desired doneness is achieved.

Beef and Broccoli Stir-Fry with Tamari Sauce

- *Serves: 4*
- *Prep time: 15 minutes.*

Ingredients:

- 1 pound beef, thinly sliced
- Four cups broccoli florets.
- 1/4 cup tamari sauce.
- Two teaspoons of sesame oil.
- 1 tablespoon minced ginger.
- 2 garlic cloves, minced
- One spoonful of cornstarch.
- One-quarter cup water

Instructions:

- In a bowl, combine the tamari sauce, sesame oil, ginger, garlic, cornstarch, and water.
- In a large skillet, heat the oil over medium-high heat. Add the steak and cook until browned.
- Add the broccoli and stir cook till tender.
- Pour the sauce over the beef and broccoli and stir until it thickens.

Stuffed Acorn Squash with Quinoa and Cranberries.

- *Serves: 4*
- *Prep time: 20 minutes.*

Ingredients:

- Two acorn squashes, halved and seeded
- 1 cup cooked quinoa.
- 1/2 cup dried cranberries.
- 1/4 cup chopped pecans.
- 1/4 cup finely chopped onion.
- One tablespoon of olive oil.
- Salt and pepper to taste.

Instructions:

- Preheat the oven to 375° F (190° C).
- Place the acorn squash halves on a baking sheet and sprinkle with olive oil. Season with salt and pepper.
- Bake for 25 minutes, or until tender.
- In a bowl, combine the cooked quinoa, cranberries, pecans, and onion.
- Stuff the quinoa mixture into the cooked squash halves and bake for an additional 10 minutes.

Chicken and Vegetable Skewers

- _**Serves: 4**_
- _**Prep time: 20 minutes, plus marinating.**_

Ingredients:

- Two chicken breasts sliced into pieces
- 1 zucchini, sliced
- 1 bell pepper, sliced into pieces
- 1 red onion, chopped into bits
- Two teaspoons of olive oil.
- Two teaspoons of tamari sauce.
- 1 clove garlic, minced
- One teaspoon of dried oregano.

Instructions:

- In a bowl, combine the olive oil, tamari sauce, garlic, and oregano.
- Thread the chicken and vegetables on skewers.
- Marinate for a minimum of 30 minutes.
- Preheat the grill to medium-high heat, then cook the skewers for 10-15 minutes, rotating periodically.

Shrimp and Asparagus Risotto

- _**Serves: 4**_
- _**Prep time: 10 minutes.**_

Ingredients:

- 1 cup arborio rice.
- 1 pound of shrimp, peeled and deveined
- 1 bunch asparagus (trimmed and chopped into bits)
- Four cups of chicken or vegetable broth.
- One-half cup white wine
- 1 onion, diced
- 2 garlic cloves, minced
- 1/4 cup grated Parmesan cheese.
- Two teaspoons of olive oil.
- Salt and pepper to taste.

Instructions:

- In a large pan, heat the olive oil over medium heat. Add the onion and garlic, and cook until transparent.
- Stir in the rice and cook for about 2 minutes, or until fully coated and opaque.
- Add the wine and simmer until the liquid is absorbed.
- Pour in the broth, one cup at a time, stirring constantly until each cup is absorbed before adding the next.

- When the rice is nearly finished, add the asparagus and shrimp. Cook until the prawns are pink and the asparagus is soft.
- Add the Parmesan cheese and season with salt and pepper.

Vegan Mushroom Stroganoff

- *Serves: 4*
- *Prep time: 10 minutes.*
- *Cook time: 15 minutes.*

Ingredients:

- One tablespoon of olive oil.
- 1 onion, diced
- 2 garlic cloves, minced
- 3 cups sliced mushrooms.
- One cup of gluten-free vegetable broth.
- 1 tablespoon of tamari (gluten-free soy sauce).
- One teaspoon Dijon mustard.
- One-half cup coconut cream
- Add salt and pepper to taste.
- Fresh parsley, chopped (to garnish)

Instructions:

- Heat the olive oil in a big pan over medium heat.
- Add the onions and garlic and sauté until transparent.
- Add the mushrooms and simmer until they release moisture and begin to brown.
- Add veggie broth and tamari and bring to a simmer.
- Add Dijon mustard and coconut cream, and heat until the sauce thickens.
- Add salt and pepper to taste.
- Serve hot and garnished with fresh parsley.

Lamb Chops with Rosemary and Garlic.

- *Serves: 4*
- *Prep time: 10 minutes.*
- *Cook time: 12 minutes.*

Ingredients:

- Eight lamb chops.
- 2 tablespoons of fresh rosemary, chopped
- 4 garlic cloves, minced
- Two teaspoons of olive oil.
- Add salt and pepper to taste.

Instructions:

- Season lamb chops with rosemary, garlic, salt, and pepper.
- Heat the olive oil in a skillet over medium-high heat.
- Add the lamb chops and cook for 3-5 minutes per side for medium-rare.
- Rest for 5 minutes before serving.

Eggplant Parmesan with Gluten-Free Breadcrumbs

- *Serves: 4*
- *Prep time: 15 minutes.*
- *Cook time: 30 minutes.*

Ingredients:

- 1 large eggplant, cut into half-inch rounds
- Salt
- Two eggs, beaten
- 1 1/2 cup gluten-free breadcrumbs.
- 1/2 cup of grated Parmesan cheese.
- 2 cups marinara sauce (gluten free)
- One cup shredded mozzarella cheese.
- Fresh basil leaves.

Instructions:

- Preheat the oven to 375° F (190° C).
- Sprinkle salt on the eggplant slices and let for 10 minutes before rinsing and patting dry.
- Dip the eggplant pieces in beaten eggs, then coat with gluten-free breadcrumbs and Parmesan cheese.
- Transfer to a baking sheet and bake for 20 minutes, flipping halfway through.
- Top each piece with marinara sauce and mozzarella cheese, then bake for another 10 minutes.
- Sprinkle with fresh basil leaves before serving.

Pork Tenderloin with Apple Cider Reduction.

- *Serves: 4*
- *Prep time: 10 minutes.*
- *Cook time: 25 minutes.*

Ingredients:

- One pork tenderloin (about one pound)
- Add salt and pepper to taste.
- One tablespoon of olive oil.
- One cup apple cider.
- One tablespoon Dijon mustard.

- One spoonful of honey.
- 2 garlic cloves, minced
- Fresh thyme.

Instructions:

- Preheat the oven to 375°F (190° C).
- Season the pork tenderloin with salt and pepper.
- Heat the olive oil in a large ovenproof skillet over medium-high heat.
- Add the pork tenderloin and cook all sides until golden brown.
- Remove the skillet from heat and place the pig in the oven.
- Roast for 15-20 minutes, until the internal temperature reaches 145°F (63°C).
- In a saucepan, whisk together apple cider, Dijon mustard, honey, and garlic while the pig roasts.
- Bring to a boil, then reduce heat and simmer until the sauce has reduced in half and thickened.
- When the pork is finished, let it rest for a few minutes before slicing and drizzling with the apple cider reduction. Garnish with fresh thyme.

Spaghetti Squash with Tomato Basil Sauce

- *Serves: 4*
- *Prep time: 10 minutes.*
- *Cook time: 40 minutes.*

Ingredients:

- One medium spaghetti squash.
- Two teaspoons of extra virgin olive oil.
- 1 onion, chopped
- 4 garlic cloves, minced
- 2 lbs ripe tomatoes, chopped
- 1/4 cup of dry red wine.
- Add salt and pepper to taste.
- Fresh basil leaves, torn

Instructions:

- Preheat your oven to 400°F (200°C).
- Cut the spaghetti squash in half lengthwise, then remove the seeds.
- Place the squash halves on a baking sheet, cut side down, and bake for about 40 minutes, or until soft.
- While the squash bakes, heat the olive oil in a large skillet over medium heat.
- Add the onion and garlic and cook until softened.

- Cook the tomatoes until they begin to break down.

- Add the wine and cook until the sauce thickens.

- Season with salt and pepper.

- When the squash is finished, use a fork to separate the flesh into strands.

- Toss the spaghetti squash with the tomato basil sauce and serve topped with fresh basil.

CHAPTER 6

Snacks And Appetizers.

Hummus With Gluten-Free Pita Chips

- *Serves: 4*
- *Prep time: 15 minutes.*

Ingredients:

- 1 can drained and rinsed chickpeas.
- 2 tablespoons tahini.
- One-quarter cup olive oil
- 2 tablespoons lemon juice.
- One clove garlic
- Salt to taste.
- Gluten-free pita bread.

Instructions:

- Using a food processor, combine the chickpeas, tahini, olive oil, lemon juice, and garlic until smooth.
- Season with salt to taste.
- Cut gluten-free pita bread into triangles and bake at 375°F until crispy, about 10-15 minutes.
- Serve the hummus with pita chips.

Caprese Salad Skewers.

- _Serves: 4_
- _Prep time: 10 minutes._

Ingredients:

- 24 cherry tomatoes.
- Twelve tiny mozzarella balls.
- Twenty-four basil leaves
- Balsamic reduction.
- Salt and pepper.

Instructions:

- Thread a tomato, a basil leaf, a mozzarella ball, another basil leaf, and another tomato on skewers.
- Drizzle with balsamic reduction, then season with salt and pepper.

Guacamole with Jicama Sticks

- _Serves: 4_
- _Prep time: 15 minutes._

Ingredients:

- Two ripe avocados.
- 1/4 cup coarsely chopped red onion.
- 1/4 cup fresh cilantro, chopped

- One lime, juiced

- Salt to taste.

- One jicama, peeled and cut into sticks

Instructions:

- Mash the avocados in a bowl.

- Add red onion, cilantro, and lime juice.

- Season with salt.

- Serve with jicama sticks for a crunchier alternative to chips.

Deviled Eggs and Avocado

- ***Servings: Six.***
- ***Prep time: 20 minutes.***

Ingredients:

- 6 hard-boiled eggs.

- One ripe avocado.

- One tablespoon of lemon juice.

- Salt and pepper.

- Paprika for garnish.

Instructions:

- Peel the eggs and cut in half lengthwise.

- Remove the yolks and combine with the avocado and lemon juice.
- Season with salt and pepper.
- Spoon or pipe the mixture back into the egg whites.
- Season with paprika before serving.

Roasted Chickpeas.

- *Serves: 4*
- *Preparation time: 5 minutes, plus 25 minutes baking.*

Ingredients:

- 1 can chickpeas (drained, rinsed, and dried)
- One tablespoon olive oil.
- 1/2 teaspoon sea salt.
- 1/2 teaspoon of garlic powder.

Instructions:

- Preheat the to 400°F.
- Toss the chickpeas with olive oil, salt, and garlic powder.
- Spread on a baking sheet and bake for approximately 25 minutes, or until crispy.

<u>*Stuffed Mushrooms*</u>

- ***Serves: 4***
- ***Preparation time: 15 minutes, plus 20 minutes baking.***

Ingredients:

- 12 big mushrooms with stems removed.
- 1/4 cup finely chopped onions.
- 2 garlic cloves, minced
- 1/4 cup of gluten-free breadcrumbs
- 1/4 cup grated parmesan cheese.
- One tablespoon olive oil.

Instructions:

- Preheat the oven to 375°F.
- Sauté the onions and garlic in olive oil until tender.
- Mix in the breadcrumbs and Parmesan cheese.
- Stuff the mixture into mushroom caps.
- Bake for 20 minutes, until the tops are golden brown.

Cucumber Rolls and Smoked Salmon

- *Serves: 4*
- *Prep time: 15 minutes.*

Ingredients:

- One large cucumber, finely sliced lengthwise.
- 4 oz smoked salmon (cut into strips)
- One-quarter cup cream cheese
- Fresh dill as garnish

Instructions

- Spread cream cheese over cucumber slices.
- Add a strip of smoked salmon to each slice.
- Roll it up and secure with a toothpick.
- Garnish with fresh dill.

Baked Kale Chips

- *Serves: 4*
- *Preparation time: 5 minutes, plus 15 minutes baking.*

Ingredients:

- 1 bunch of kale, stems removed and torn into bite-sized pieces.

- One tablespoon olive oil.

- Salt to taste.

Instructions:

- Preheat the oven to 350°F.

- Toss greens with olive oil and salt.

- Spread out on a baking sheet and bake for 15 minutes, or until the edges are crispy.

Almond Butter And Banana On Rice Cakes

- ***Serves: 4***

- ***Prep time: 5 minutes.***

Ingredients:

- Four rice cakes.

- Four tablespoons almond butter.

- Two bananas, cut

- Cinnamon to sprinkle.

Instructions:

- Spread almond butter over rice cakes.

- Top with banana slices.

- Sprinkle with cinnamon.

Gluten-Free Bruschetta.

- *Serves: 4*
- *Prep time: 10 minutes plus chilling.*

Ingredients:

- Dice three Roma tomatoes.
- 1 clove garlic, minced
- 1 teaspoon of olive oil.
- 1 1/2 teaspoons balsamic vinegar.
- 1/4 cup fresh basil, minced
- Salt and pepper.
- Gluten-free crackers or toasted bread.

Instructions:

- In a bowl, combine tomatoes, garlic, olive oil, balsamic vinegar, and basil.
- Season with salt and pepper.
- Allow to chill for at least an hour.
- Serve with gluten-free crackers or toasted bread.

CHAPTER 7

Flourless Chocolate Cake

- *Servings: 8–10.*
- *Prep time: 20 minutes.*

Ingredients:

- 1 cup semisweet chocolate chips (gluten free)
- 1/2 cup of unsalted butter.
- 3/4 cup granulated sugar.
- 1/4 teaspoon of salt.
- One teaspoon of vanilla extract.
- Three big eggs.
- 1/2 cup unsweetened cocoa powder, gluten-free

Instructions:

- Preheat the oven to 375°F (190° C). Grease an 8-inch cake pan and line with parchment paper.
- Heat the chocolate chips and butter in a double boiler or microwave, stirring until smooth.
- Stir in the sugar, salt, and vanilla extract.

- Add the eggs one at a time, beating thoroughly after each addition.
- Sift in cocoa powder and stir until just mixed.
- Transfer the batter to the prepared pan and bake for 25 minutes.
- Let cool in the pan for 5 minutes before inverting onto a platter.

Baked Apples with Cinnamon.

- *Serves: 4*
- *Prep time: 15 minutes.*

Ingredients:

- Four big, cored apples
- 4 tablespoons of unsalted butter (or coconut oil if dairy-free).
- Two teaspoons of ground cinnamon.
- 1/4 cup maple syrup.

Instructions:

- Preheat the oven to 350°F/175°C.
- Place the apples in a baking dish.
- Fill each apple with a spoonful of butter and top with cinnamon.
- Drizzle maple syrup over the apples.

- Bake for 30 to 40 minutes, or until the apples are soft.

Almond Flour Blueberry Muffins.

- *Servings: 12 muffins.*
- *Prep time: 15 minutes.*

Ingredients:

- Two cups almond flour.
- 1/2 teaspoon of baking soda.
- A pinch of salt.
- 1/4 cup honey or maple syrup.
- Two big eggs.
- 1/4 cup of unsweetened almond milk.
- One teaspoon of vanilla extract.
- One cup of fresh blueberries

Instructions:

- Preheat the oven to 325°F (165° C). Line the muffin tray with paper liners.
- In a bowl, combine almond flour, baking soda, and salt.
- In another bowl, combine the honey, eggs, almond milk, and vanilla essence.
- Combine wet and dry ingredients and fold in blueberries.
- Scoop batter into muffin cups and bake for 20-25 minutes.

Coconut Macaroons.

- *Serving size: 15 macaroons.*
- *Prep time: 10 minutes.*

Ingredients:

- 2 1/2 cups unsweetened, shredded coconut
- 3/4 cup granulated sugar.
- Two big egg whites.
- One teaspoon of vanilla extract.
- A pinch of salt.

Instructions:

- Preheat the oven to 325°F (165° C). Line a baking sheet with parchment paper.
- In a mixing basin, combine all of the ingredients thoroughly.
- Transfer spoonful of the mixture on the baking sheet.
- Bake for 15-20 minutes, until golden brown.

Gluten-Free Lemon Bars

- *Servings: nine bars.*
- *Prep time: 20 minutes.*

Ingredients:

• *For the crust:*

- 1/2 cup unsalted butter, melted
- 1 cup gluten-free flour mixture.
- 1/4 cup powdered sugar.

• *For the Filling:*

- 1 1/2 cups granulated sugar.
- 1/4 cup gluten-free flour mixture.
- Four big eggs.
- 2/3 cup fresh lemon juice.
- One tablespoon of lemon zest.

Instructions:

- Preheat the oven to 350°F/175°C. Line an 8-by-8-inch baking pan with parchment paper.
- Combine the crust ingredients and press onto the bottom of the pan. Bake for fifteen minutes.
- Whisk together the filling ingredients and pour over the cooked crust.

- Bake for a further 20 to 25 minutes. Let cool before cutting into bars.

Chocolate Avocado Pudding.

- *Serves: 4*
- *Prep time: 10 minutes.*

Ingredients:

- Two ripe avocados, peeled and pitted.
- 1/4 cup cocoa powder, gluten-free.
- 1/4 cup honey or maple syrup.
- One-half cup coconut milk
- One teaspoon of vanilla extract.

Instructions:

- Using a food processor, combine all ingredients until smooth.
- Refrigerate for at least one hour before serving.

Raspberry Sorbet

- ***Servings: Six.***
- ***Preparation time: 10 minutes (including freezing time).***

Ingredients:

- 4 cups fresh raspberries.
- 3/4 cup granulated sugar.
- One cup of water.
- 2 teaspoons of lemon juice.

Instructions:

- Puree raspberries in a blender, then filter to remove seeds.
- In a saucepan, melt sugar in water over medium heat. Add lemon juice.
- Combine the syrup and raspberry puree and freeze in an ice cream maker according to the manufacturer's directions.

<u>*Peanut Butter Cookies.*</u>

- ***Serving size: 24 cookies.***
- ***Prep time: 15 minutes.***

Ingredients:

- 1 cup natural peanut butter (gluten free)
- One cup granulated sugar.
- One big egg.
- One teaspoon of baking soda.

Instructions:

- Preheat the oven to 350°F/175°C. Line a baking sheet with parchment paper.
- Mix all of the ingredients together until thoroughly blended.
- Form dough into balls and lay them on the baking pan. Flatten using a fork.
- Bake for 10-12 minutes, until golden brown.

Poached Pear with White Wine.

- *Serves: 4*
- *Prep time: 10 minutes.*

Ingredients:

- Four ripe, peeled pears
- One bottle of white wine
- 1/2 cup granulated sugar.
- One vanilla bean, split
- One cinnamon stick.

Instructions:

- In a large pot, combine the wine, sugar, vanilla bean, and cinnamon sticks. Bring to a simmer.
- Add the pears and cook for 15-20 minutes, until tender.
- Drizzle pears with the poaching liquid.

Pumpkin Pie with Gluten-free Crust

- *Servings: eight.*
- *Prep time: 20 minutes.*

Ingredients:

• *For the crust:*

- 1 1/4 cups gluten-free flour mixture

- 1/2 cup cold, unsalted butter, cubed

- 1/4 teaspoon of salt.

- 2-4 teaspoons of ice water.

• *For the Filling:*

- One (15-ounce) can of pumpkin puree

- 3/4 cup granulated sugar.

- 1/2 teaspoon of salt.

- One teaspoon of ground cinnamon.

- 1/2 teaspoon of ground ginger.

- 1/4 teaspoon of ground cloves.

- Two big eggs.

- 1 (12-ounce) can of evaporated milk.

Instructions:

- Preheat the oven to 425°F (220°C).

- In a food processor, combine flour, butter, and salt until crumbly. Add ice water until the dough forms.

- Place the dough in a 9-inch pie dish and bake for 8 minutes.

- Combine the filling ingredients and pour into the crust.

- Bake for 15 minutes, then lower the heat to 350°F (175°C) and bake for 40-50 minutes.

<u>*2-Week Meal Plan*</u>

Week 1

Day 1:

- Breakfast: Quinoa porridge with mixed berries.
- Lunch: Quinoa salad with roasted vegetables.
- Dinner is grilled salmon with lemon and dill.
- Snack 1: Hummus and Gluten-Free Pita Chips
- Snack 2: Almond Butter and Banana on Rice Cakes
- Dessert: Flourless chocolate cake.

Day 2:

- Breakfast: Buckwheat Pancakes with Maple Syrup
- Lunch is Buckwheat Soba Noodle Salad.
- Dinner: Stir-Fried Beef and Broccoli with Tamari Sauce
- Snack 1: Caprese Salad Skewers
- Snack 2: Baked Kale Chips
- Dessert: Baked apples with cinnamon.

Day 3:

- Breakfast: Chia Seed Pudding and Almond Milk
- Lunch is grilled chicken breast with avocado and mango salsa.
- Dinner is Stuffed Acorn Squash with Quinoa and Cranberries.
- Snack 1: Guacamole and Jicama Sticks.
- Snack 2: Roasted Chickpeas
- Dessert: Almond Flour Blueberry Muffins.

Day 4:

- Breakfast: Smoothie bowl with spinach, avocado, and banana.
- Lunch: Lentil soup with carrots and celery.
- Dinner: Chicken and vegetable skewers
- Snack 1: Devilled eggs and avocado.
- Snack 2: Stuffed Mushrooms
- Dessert: coconut macaroons.

Day 5:

- Breakfast: Baked Amaranth with Almond Milk
- Lunch: Baked falafel with Tahini Sauce.
- Dinner: Shrimp and asparagus risotto.
- Snack 1: Cucumber Rolls with Smoked Salmon

- Snack 2: Gluten-free Bruschetta
- Dessert: Gluten-free Lemon Bars.

Day 6:

- Breakfast: Gluten-free oats with cinnamon and apple.
- Lunch: Stuffed bell peppers with ground turkey and herbs.
- Dinner is Vegan Mushroom Stroganoff.
- Snack 1: Baked Kale Chips
- Snack 2: Almond Butter and Banana on Rice Cakes
- Dessert is Chocolate Avocado Pudding.

Day 7:

- Breakfast: Baked sweet potatoes with yogurt and nuts.
- Lunch: Stir-fried Cauliflower Rice with Mixed Vegetables
- Dinner: Lamb chops with rosemary and garlic.
- Snack 1: Hummus and Gluten-Free Pita Chips
- Snack 2: Caprese Salad Skewers.
- Dessert: raspberry sorbet.

Week 2

Day 8:

- Breakfast: Savoury Vegetable Muffins
- Lunch: Spinach and goat cheese frittata.
- Dinner: Eggplant Parmesan with gluten-free breadcrumbs.
- Snack 1: Guacamole and Jicama Sticks.
- Snack 2: Roasted Chickpeas
- Dessert: Peanut butter cookies.

Day 9:

- Breakfast: Coconut yogurt with gluten-free granola.
- Lunch: Zucchini noodles with pesto and cherry tomatoes.
- Dinner: Pork tenderloin with apple cider reduction.
- Snack 1: Devilled eggs and avocado.
- Snack 2: Stuffed Mushrooms
- Dessert: poached pears in white wine.

Day 10:

- Breakfast: egg white omelette with spinach and mushrooms.
- Lunch: Turkey and Spinach Wraps with Gluten-Free Tortillas
- Dinner is spaghetti squash with tomato basil sauce.

- Snack 1: Cucumber Rolls with Smoked Salmon

- Snack 2: Gluten-free Bruschetta

- Dessert: Pumpkin pie with gluten-free crust.

Day 11:

- Breakfast: Quinoa porridge with mixed berries.

- Lunch: Quinoa salad with roasted vegetables.

- Dinner is grilled salmon with lemon and dill.

- Snack 1: Hummus and Gluten-Free Pita Chips

- Snack 2: Almond Butter and Banana on Rice Cakes

- Dessert: Flourless chocolate cake.

Day 12:

- Breakfast: Buckwheat Pancakes with Maple Syrup

- Lunch is Buckwheat Soba Noodle Salad.

- Dinner: Stir-Fried Beef and Broccoli with Tamari Sauce

- Snack 1: Caprese Salad Skewers

- Snack 2: Baked Kale Chips

- Dessert: Baked apples with cinnamon.

Day 13:

- Breakfast: Chia Seed Pudding and Almond Milk

- Lunch is grilled chicken breast with avocado and mango salsa.

- Dinner is Stuffed Acorn Squash with Quinoa and Cranberries.
- Snack 1: Guacamole and Jicama Sticks.
- Snack 2: Roasted Chickpeas
- Dessert: Almond Flour Blueberry Muffins.

Day 14:

- Breakfast: Smoothie bowl with spinach, avocado, and banana.
- Lunch: Lentil soup with carrots and celery.
- Dinner: Chicken and vegetable skewers
- Snack 1: Devilled eggs and avocado.
- Snack 2: Stuffed Mushrooms
- Dessert: coconut macaroons.

Enjoy two weeks of wonderful gluten-free meals!

CONCLUSION

As we come to the end of our culinary journey, I hope that the recipes and thoughts provided have not only piqued your interest, but also paved the way to a healthy, gluten-free living.

Adopting a gluten-free gut health diet is more than just a matter of ingredients; it is a commitment to feeding your body and meeting its requirements. Consistency is essential, and each meal brings you closer to being a more vibrant and energetic version of yourself.

Remember that, while this book can help you eat deliciously and nutritiously, you should always seek personalized guidance from a healthcare practitioner.

Your unique health profile requires personalized care, and a nutritionist or doctor can make tailored recommendations to ensure that your food choices are in line with your health goals.

If this book has expanded your culinary palette and improved your overall well-being, I would appreciate it if you could share your positive experiences. Your positive feedback is not only a source of encouragement, but also a compass that helps others on their journey to health and happiness. Please consider writing Positive Feedback or sharing your opinions on this book with others who may be on a similar journey.

Thank you for inviting me to take part in your gluten-free journey.

May Your Meals Be as Enjoyable as They Are Nutritious, And May Your Journey Be Filled with The Riches of Good Health and The Pleasure of Well-Being.